Table of Contents

Introduction...5

    What is the Fasting Mimicking Diet?...................7

    How does it work?....................................7

Foods to eat and to avoid...................................9

    What are the benefits?..............................12

    Who should avoid the fasting mimicking diet? 16

Recipes 19

    Blood Orange Cabbage Salad 19

    Sauteed Carrots and Parsnips with Honey and Rosemary20

    Spaghetti Squash with Basil-Parsley Pesto and Sauteed Shrimp..21

    Ginger and Turmeric Aromatic Rice...................24

    Oven Roasted Chickpeas with Caramelized Bananas and Cavolo Nero 26

    Spiced Apple Carrot Muffin..........................27

    The Ultimate Detox Salad............................29

    Strawberry Gazpacho.................................31

    Chocolate Superfood Smoothie........................32

Overnight Oats 33

Banana Blueberry Ice Cream 34

Strawberry Banana Beet Ice Cream 36

Moroccan Chickpea and Vegetable Tagine 37

Raw Vegan Pecan Pie 39

Quinoa Lentil Pumpkin Salad 41

Farmer's Market Salad 42

Poached Halibut with Sweet Garlic, Parsley, and Lemon . 44

Raw Cauliflower Couscous with Kale and Cabbage 46

Mushroom with Lentils 47

Avocado Tofu Salad with Ponzu Recipe 49

Pesto with Walnuts 50

Black Risotto 51

Quinoa Carrot Cakes 54

Arugula and Lentil Salad with Strawberry-Balsamic Dressing

.... 56

Creamy Mango and Rhubarb Smoothie 58

Zesty Orange and Carrot Smoothie 59

Roasted baby cauliflower, fried coriander chickpeas, caper dressing, crushed pistachio and greek yogurt 60

Eat to Beat Brownies...62

Indian Spiced Tomato Soup...64

Spiced Chocolate Mousse 66

Baked Tarragon Oil & Lemon Fish with Kale Pesto Quinoa 67

Roasted Spiced Chickpeas Over Kale Caesar Salad.........68

Roasted Beet Pesto...71

Sweet Potato Apple Soup 72

Pecan, Granny Smith & Kale salad 74

Sweet Potato and Turnip Mash with Fresh Sage 75

Sauteed Chicken Breast with Kale and Wild Mushrooms .77

Introduction

Fasting is a hot topic in health and wellness, and for good reason.

It's been associated with a wide range of benefits — from weight loss to boosting your body's health and life span.

There are many types of fasting methods, such as intermittent fasting and water fasting.

"Fast Mimicking" is a recent fasting trend that restricts calories for a set time period.

This guide reviews the Fasting Mimicking Diet, so you can decide whether it's right for you.

DIET REVIEW SCORECARD

Overall score: 2.88

Weight loss: 3.75

Healthy eating: 2.5

Sustainability: 2.5

Whole body health: 2

Nutrition quality: 3.5

Evidence based: 3

BOTTOM LINE: The Fasting Mimicking Diet is a high-fat, low-calorie intermittent fasting method that supplies prepackaged meals for five days. It may help you lose weight but is pricey and may not be better than standard intermittent fasting diets.

What is the Fasting Mimicking Diet?

The Fasting Mimicking Diet was created by Dr. Valter Longo, an Italian biologist and researcher.

He sought to replicate the benefits of fasting while still providing the body with nutrition. His modifications avoid the calorie deprivation associated with other types of fasting.

The Fasting Mimicking Diet — or "fast mimicking" — is a type of intermittent fasting. However, it differs from more traditional types, such as the 16/8 method.

The Fasting Mimicking protocol is based on decades of research, including several clinical studies.

How does it work?

The ProLon Fasting Mimicking Diet plan includes five-day, prepackaged meal kits.

All meals and snacks are whole-food derived and plant based. The meal kits are low in carbs and protein yet high in healthy fats like olives and flax.

During the five-day period, dieters only consume what's contained within the meal kit.

Day one of the diet provides approximately 1,090 kcal (10% protein, 56% fat, 34% carbs), while days two through five provide only 725 kcal (9% protein, 44% fat, 47% carbs).

The low-calorie, high-fat, low-carb content of the meals causes your body to generate energy from noncarbohydrate sources after glycogen stores are depleted. This process is called gluconeogenesis.

According to one study, the diet is designed to provide 34–54% of normal calorie intake.

This calorie restriction mimics the body's physiological response to traditional fasting methods, such as cell regeneration, decreased inflammation, and fat loss.

ProLon recommends that all dieters consult a medical professional — such as a doctor or registered dietitian — before starting the five-day fast.

The ProLon five-day plan is not a one-time cleanse and must be followed every one to six months to obtain optimal results.

SUMMARY

The ProLon Fasting Mimicking Diet is a low-calorie, five-day eating program meant to promote weight loss and provide the same benefits as more traditional fasting methods.

Foods to eat and to avoid

The ProLon meal kit is broken down into five individual boxes — one box per day — and includes a chart with recommendations on what foods to eat and the order in which to eat them.

A specific combination of food is provided for breakfast, lunch, dinner, and snacks, depending on the day.

The unique combination of nutrients and reduction in calories is meant to trick your body into thinking it's fasting, even though it's being given energy.

Because calories vary between days, it's important that dieters do not mix foods or carry foods over into the next day.

All foods are vegetarian, as well as gluten- and lactose-free. The purchased kit comes with nutritional facts.

A five-day ProLon Fasting Mimicking Diet kit includes:

Nut bars. Meal bars made from macadamia nut butter, honey, flax, almond meal, and coconut.

Algal oil. A vegetarian-based supplement that provide dieters with 200 mg of the omega-3 fatty acid DHA.

Soup blends. A mix of flavored soups including minestrone, minestrone quinoa, mushroom, and tomato soup.

Herbal tea. Spearmint, hibiscus, and lemon-spearmint tea.

Dark chocolate crisp bar. A dessert bar made with cocoa powder, almonds, chocolate chips, and flax.

Kale crackers. A mix of ingredients including flax seeds, nutritional yeast, kale, herbs, and pumpkin seeds.

Olives. Olives are included as a high-fat snack. One pack is provided on day one, while two packs are provided on days two through five.

NR-1. A powdered vegetable supplement that delivers a dose of vitamins and minerals that you wouldn't normally consume during a traditional fast.

L-Drink. This glycerol-based energy drink is given on days two through five when your body has started gluconeogenesis (begins to create energy from noncarbohydrate sources, such as fats).

Dieters are encouraged to only consume what is contained within the meal kit and to avoid consuming any other foods or beverages with two exceptions:

Soups can be flavored with fresh herbs and lemon juice.

Dieters are encouraged to stay hydrated with plain water and decaffeinated teas during the five-day fast.

SUMMARY

The ProLon meal kit contains soups, olives, herbal teas, nut bars, nutritional supplements, chocolate bars, and energy drinks. Dieters are encouraged to only eat these items during their five-day fast.

What are the benefits?

Unlike the majority of diets on the market, the ProLon Fasting Mimicking Diet is supported by research.

Plus, multiple research studies have demonstrated the health benefits of similar fasting methods.

May promote weight loss

A small study led by Dr. Longo compared people who completed three cycles of the ProLon Fasting Mimicking Diet over three months to a control group.

Participants in the fasting group lost an average of 6 pounds (2.7 kg) and experienced greater reductions in belly fat than the control group.

Though this study was small and led by the developer of the ProLon Fasting Mimicking Diet, other studies have shown that fasting methods are effective in promoting weight loss.

For example, one 16-week study in obese men found that those who practiced intermittent fasting lost 47% more weight than those who continuously restricted calories.

What's more, very-low-calorie diets have been proven to encourage weight loss.

Still, evidence that the ProLon Fasting Mimicking Diet is more effective than other low-calorie diets or fasting methods is currently lacking.

May reduce blood sugar and cholesterol levels

The same small study led by Dr. Longo that linked fast mimicking to fat loss also observed that the Fasting Mimicking Diet group experienced a significant drop in blood sugar and cholesterol levels.

Cholesterol was reduced by 20 mg/dl in those with high cholesterol levels, while blood sugar levels dropped into the normal range in participants who had high blood sugar at the beginning of the study.

These results were also demonstrated in animal studies.

Four days of the diet every week for 60 days prompted regeneration of damaged pancreatic cells, promoted healthy insulin production, reduced insulin resistance, and led to more stable levels of blood glucose in mice with diabetes.

Although these results are promising, more human studies are needed to determine the diet's impact on blood sugar.

May reduce inflammation

Studies have shown that intermittent fasting reduces markers of inflammation, such as C-reactive protein (CRP), tumor necrosis factor-alpha (TNF-α), interferon gamma (ifnγ), leptin, interleukin 1 beta (IL-1β), and interleukin 6 (IL-6).

In a study in people practicing alternate-day fasting for the religious holiday of Ramadan, proinflammatory cytokines were significantly lower during the alternate-day fasting period, compared to the weeks before or after.

One animal study found that the Fasting Mimicking Diet may be effective at reducing certain inflammatory markers.

Mice with multiple sclerosis were placed on either the Fasting Mimicking Diet or a ketogenic diet for 30 days.

The mice in the fasting group had significantly lower levels of ifnγ and the T helper cells Th1 and Th17 — proinflammatory cells associated with autoimmune disease.

May slow aging and mental decline

One of the main reasons Dr. Longo developed the Fasting Mimicking Diet was to slow the aging process and risk of certain diseases by promoting the body's ability to self-repair through cellular regeneration.

Autophagy is a process in which old, damaged cells are recycled to produce new, healthier ones.

Intermittent fasting has been shown to optimize autophagy, which may protect against mental decline and slow cellular aging.

A study in mice found that short-term food restriction led to a dramatic increase of autophagy in nerve cells.

Another study in rats with dementia showed that alternate-day food deprivation for 12 weeks led to greater reductions in oxidative damage to brain tissue and reduced mental deficits compared to a control diet.

Other animal studies have demonstrated that fasting increases the generation of nerve cells and enhances brain function.

What's more, intermittent fasting has been shown to decrease insulin-like growth factor (IGF-1) — a hormone that, at high levels, can increase the risk of certain cancer, such as breast cancer.

However, more human studies need to be carried out to fully understand how fasting may impact aging and disease risk.

SUMMARY

The Fasting Mimicking Diet may promote weight loss, enhance autophagy, and reduce blood sugar, cholesterol, and inflammation.

Who should avoid the fasting mimicking diet?

ProLon does not recommend its diet to certain populations, such as pregnant or breastfeeding women and those who are underweight or malnourished.

People who are allergic to nuts, soy, oats, sesame, or celery/celeriac should also avoid the ProLon meal kit as it contains these ingredients.

Additionally, ProLon warns anyone with medical conditions — such as diabetes or kidney disease — to only use the plan under a doctor's supervision.

Intermittent fasting may also not be appropriate for those with a history of disordered eating.

SUMMARY

Pregnant or breastfeeding women, and those with allergies and certain medical conditions should avoid this diet.

Should you try it?

The Fasting Mimicking Diet is most likely safe for healthy individuals and may provide several health benefits.

However, it's unclear whether it's more effective than other, more researched methods of intermittent fasting, such as the 16/8 method.

The 16/8 method is a type of intermittent fasting that limits eating to eight hours per day, with no food for the remaining 16 hours. This cycle can be repeated once or twice per week or every day, depending on personal preference.

If you have the funds and the self-discipline to follow the five-day, low-calorie fasting plan from ProLon, it may be a good choice.

Just remember that — like other fasting methods — this diet needs to be continued long term to reap the potential benefits.

It's possible to fast mimic without using the ProLon prepackaged meal kit.

Those with nutrition knowledge can create their own high-fat, low-carb, low-protein, calorie-controlled, five-day meal plan.

Some fast mimicking meal plans are available online but they don't deliver the same nutrition as the ProLon meal kit — which may be the key to the diet's effectiveness.

For those interested in trying intermittent fasting, a more researched, cost-effective plan, like the 16/8 method, may be a better choice.

SUMMARY

For those interested in intermittent fasting, the 16/8 method may be a more cost-effective choice than ProLon.

The bottom line

The ProLon Fasting Mimicking Diet is a high-fat, low-calorie intermittent fasting diet that may promote fat loss and reduce blood sugar, inflammation, and cholesterol — similar to other fasting methods.

Still, only one human study has been carried out to date, and more research is needed to validate its benefits.

Recipes

Blood Orange Cabbage Salad

Serves 4, as a salad course

Ingredients:

- 2 carrots
- 1 purple cabbage
- 5 radishes
- 2 blood oranges
- golden raisins
- olive oil
- balsamic vinegar
- juice of 1 blood orange

1. Slice or chop 2 carrots, 1 purple cabbage, 5 radishes and 2 blood oranges. Toss together with a handful of golden raisins. Make a simple dressing of olive oil, balsamic vinegar and the juice from one more blood orange. Use a couple of the outer cabbage leaves as bowls for a pretty look. A wintery citrusy delight!

Sauteed Carrots and Parsnips with Honey and Rosemary

Serves 8, as a side course

Ingredients:

- 2 Tbsp extra virgin olive oil
- 1 lb large carrots (about 4), peeled and quartered into 4 inch sticks
- 1 lb parsnips, peeled, halved lengthwise, cored, and cut into 4 inch sticks
- Coarse salt such as Sel de Guérande (or Kosher salt)
- Black pepper, freshly ground
- 1 Tbsp butter
- 1 Tbsp fresh rosemary leaves, stripped from branches, and chopped
- 2 Tbsp honey (such as chestnut, heather, or wildflower)
- Optional: 1/4 cup chopped, toasted walnuts

Directions:

1. Heat oil in a large skillet over medium-high heat. Add carrots and saute for a few minutes before adding parsnips. Stir often until vegetables are beginning to

brown at edges, about 12 minutes. Season with salt and pepper. Vegetables can be made ahead and reserved at this point, if desired.

2. Just prior to serving, add butter, rosemary, and honey to skillet with vegetables, and toss over medium heat until glazed and heated through.

3. Sprinkle with chopped walnuts, if using, just before serving.

Spaghetti Squash with Basil-Parsley Pesto and Sauteed Shrimp

Serves 3-4, as a main course

Ingredients:

- 1 4-pound spaghetti squash
- 1 to 2 tablespoons olive oil
- Salt and pepper

Basil-Parsley Pesto Sauce:

- ½ cup tightly packed basil leaves
- ½ cup tightly packed parsley leaves
- 2 cloves garlic, minced

- 1/3 cup pine nuts
- ¼ teaspoon salt, or to taste
- ½ cup olive oil or grapeseed oil

For the Shrimp:

- 1 pound raw shrimp, peeled and deveined
- 2 tablespoons olive oil
- 3 cloves garlic, minced

For Serving:

- pine nuts
- Lemon wedges
- Parmesan cheese

Directions:

Roast the Spaghetti Squash:

1. Preheat the oven to 400 degrees F.
2. Chop the tip and the tail off of the spaghetti squash, and stand the squash up-right on a cutting board. Carefully cut the squash in half length-wise - gravity will help you chop from top to bottom.
3. Use a spoon to scoop the seeds out of each of the halves.

4. Rub about a tablespoon of olive oil over the flesh of each half. Sprinkle generously with salt and pepper.

5. Place both halves cut-side down on a baking sheet.

6. Roast the squash for 45 to 50 minutes or until the flesh is tender. Remove from oven and allow squash to cool about 10 minutes.

7. When the squash is cool enough to handle, use a fork to gently scrape the flesh, releasing spaghetti-like stands. Do this until both halves of the spaghetti squash are scraped clean and place the "spaghetti" into a large serving bowl and set aside.

Prepare the Basil-Parsley Pesto Sauce:

1. Add all ingredients for the pesto sauce to a small blender (or food processor) and blend until it reaches desired consistency. I blended mine until smooth.

Sauté the Shrimp:

1. In a large skillet, heat the oil to medium.

2. Carefully place the shrimp on the hot skillet, and add the garlic.

3. Allow shrimp to cook until it begins to plump and turn pink, about 1 to 2 minutes.

4. Flip shrimp to the other side and allow it to cook an additional 1 to 2 minutes, or until cooked through.

5. Lower the heat to medium-low, and add the pesto sauce and prepared spaghetti squash. Fold everything together and cook until everything is hot.

6. Serve heaping portions with pine nuts, fresh lemon wedges, and grated parmesan cheese.

Ginger and Turmeric Aromatic Rice

Serves , as a side course

Ingredients:

- 1 cup basmati brown rice
- 1 tablespoon coconut oil or oil of choice
- 2 large cloves garlic, minced
- 1 tablespoon ginger, peeled and grated
- 1 teaspoon turmeric, peeled and grated*
- ¾ teaspoon salt
- 2 cups boiling water
- 1 tablespoon fresh lemon juice
- ½ cup dried cranberries

For serving:

- ¼ cup fresh cilantro, chopped
- ¼ cup pine nuts

Directions:

1. Pour the dry rice into a bowl and cover with cool water. Soak for 15 minutes, then drain.
2. While rice is soaking, put on a kettle of water and bring to a full boil.
3. Add the coconut oil, garlic, and ginger to a medium-sized pot and heat to medium. Sauté until very fragrant, about 3 minutes.
4. Add the rice, turmeric and salt, and sauté an additional 2 to 3 minutes.
5. Add 2 cups of boiling water, reduce heat and simmer, covered until water is absorbed, about 30 to 35 minutes.
6. A few minutes before rice is finished cooking, stir the fresh lemon juice and dried cranberries into the rice. Re-place the cover and continue to cook.
7. Serve with fresh cilantro and pine nuts alongside your favorite main dish.

Oven Roasted Chickpeas with Caramelized Bananas and Cavolo Nero

Serves 2, as a side course

Ingredients:

- 1 tin chickpeas, drained
- 1 small red onion, roughly chopped
- 2 ripe bananas, sliced
- 1 tablespoon curry powder
- 1 teaspoon coriander seeds (optional jazz)
- 2-3 tablespoons extra virgin coconut or olive oil
- 1 bunch cavolo nero (type of cabbage)

Directions:

1. Fire up your oven to 200 Celsius /180 fan-assisted. Let it get really hot while you prep the supper.
2. Toss the chickpeas, red onion and banana discs onto your largest roasting tray and coat with the spices and preferred oil. Curry powders can vary wildly, so add a pinch of luminous turmeric powder if you fancy a healthy neon glow. I do.
3. Roast for 15 minutes, or until the banana looks caramelised and the chickpeas are turning crispy. If

your roasting tray is small, everything will sweat and turn soggy instead of caramelising so it might be worth spreading over two small trays.

4. While the chickpeas are raving in the oven, tear the green parts of the cavolo nero off its tough stalk. Gently rip into bite-sized pieces, and tumble into the hot chickpeas. You might need an extra splash of olive oil if everything looks dry. Return to the oven for 3 minutes.

Spiced Apple Carrot Muffin

Serves , as a course

Ingredients:

- 1 large carrot, peeled and grated (1.5 cups shredded carrot)]
- 1 Fuji apple, peeled and grated
- 2 eggs, lightly beaten
- 1/3 cup coconut milk
- 3 tablespoons pure maple syrup
- 1 teaspoon fresh ginger, peeled and grated
- ¼ cup almond meal

- ¾ cup brown rice flour
- 1 tablespoon baking powder
- 1 teaspoon ground cinnamon
- 1/8 teaspoon ground nutmeg
- ¼ teaspoon kosher salt

Instructions

1. Preheat the oven to 375 degrees F and lightly oil a 9-hole muffin pan
2. Whisk together the eggs, coconut milk, maple syrup, and ginger.
3. Add in the grated carrot and apple and stir to combine.
4. In a separate bowl, mix together the remaining (dry) ingredients.
5. Pour the dry ingredients into the bowl with the wet ingredients and mix until combined.
6. Fill the muffin holes 3/4 of the way up and bake for 20 to 25 minutes, or until muffins test clean.

The Ultimate Detox Salad

Serves 6, as a lunch or dinner course

Ingredients:

For the dressing:

- 1/3 cup grapeseed oil
- 1/2 cup lemon juice, fresh
- 1 tablespoon ginger, peeled and grated
- 2 teaspoons whole grain mustard
- 2 teaspoons pure maple syrup, optional
- 1/4 teaspoon salt, or to taste

For the salad:

- 2 cups dinosaur kale, tightly packed and thinly sliced
- 2 cups red cabbage, thinly sliced
- 2 cups broccoli florets
- 2 large carrots, peeled and grated
- 1 red bell pepper, sliced into matchsticks
- 2 avocados, peeled and diced
- 1/2 cup fresh parsley, chopped
- 1 cup walnuts
- 1 tablespoon sesame seeds

Directions

1. Whisk together all ingredients for the dressing (or put everything in a small blender and blend) and set aside until ready to use.
2. Add the kale, cabbage, broccoli, bell pepper, and carrots to a large serving bowl.
3. Pour desired amount of dressing over the salad and toss until everything is coated.
4. Add the parsley, diced avocado, sesame seeds and walnuts and toss again.
5. Serve as an entrée salad or as a side salad to your favorite meal.

Notes

• I used dinosaur kale, but you can use any type of kale you like.

• You can also use avocado oil or olive oil in place of grapeseed oil in the dressing.

Strawberry Gazpacho

Serves 5, as a lunch course

Ingredients:

- 2 cloves garlic, peeled and crushed
- 1 small punnet / 250g baby tomatoes, quartered
- Handful of strawberries, greens removed
- 1 red pepper, de-seeded and diced
- 1 cup finely diced cucumber
- 3 spring onions, sliced
- 2 -3 cups / 500 – 700ml tomato passata
- Juice of 1 large lemon
- Fresh crack of black pepper
- ¼ teaspoon smoked paprika powder
- ¼ teaspoon cayenne pepper
- Basil leaves to decorate
- Extra virgin olive oil to serve

Directions:

1. Using a high-speed blender, blitz the garlic with your tomatoes and strawberries. Add in the remaining ingredients (excluding your olive oil and basil) and puree until smooth. If your lemon was huge, you may

need to add a touch of maple syrup to balance the sharpness.

2. Chill in the refrigerator for at least 2 hours before spooning into five shallow soup bowls. Should the gazpacho seems too thick or separate in layers, give it another belt in the food processor before pouring into bowls. Tickle with fruity olive oil, ice cubes and a few basil leaves.

Radically fabulous.

Chocolate Superfood Smoothie

Serves 1, as a dessert course

Ingredients:

- 1 cup coconut water (or filtered water | tea | spring water)
- 1 banana (or 2 if you want smoothie to be thicker)
- 1 tsp cacao nibs
- 1 tsp organic cacao powder
- 1 tsp cacao butter
- 1 cup (or 2) of berries: blueberries, raspberries, strawberries

- 1 handful of soaked cashews (or cashew butter | almond butter)
- 1 tsp maca
- 1 tsp hemp seeds
- 1 tsp spirulina
- goji berries for topping or any frozen berries (I chose raspberries!)

Directions:

1. Simply blend everything together!

Overnight Oats

Serves 2, as a breakfast course

Ingredients:

- 1 cup rolled oats (not quick oats)
- 1 cup milk of choice (soy, regular, coconut, almond)
- 1/2 cup Greek yogurt
- 1-2 Tbs agave or honey
- 1/2 tsp cinnamon
- 1/2 tsp chia seeds
- tiny pinch of salt
- 2 Tbs shredded coconut

- 2 Tbs chopped walnuts
- 3 medjool dried dates cut into small pieces
- Fresh fruit (bananas, or peaches) for topping

Directions:

1. Place everything except the fresh fruit in a lidded container or jar. Mix together and cover. Place in fridge over night or for a few hours at a minimum.
2. In the morning, check the consistency and add a little more milk if desired and top with fresh fruit and/or nuts.

Banana Blueberry Ice Cream

Serves 1, as a dessert course

Ingredients:

- 1 – 2 frozen bananas depending on size (freeze when very ripe)
- 1/2 cup frozen blueberries
- Unsweetened vanilla almond milk, enough to blend
- Splash sweetener, if desired
- Hemp hearts
- Chia Seeds

- Unsweetened coconut flakes

Directions:

1. Slice very ripe bananas and place in freezer along with the blueberries, preferably overnight.
2. Pour a generous splash of the almond milk into the blender (you will need to use more if you are not using a high speed blender). Throw in the frozen bananas and blueberries and blend until you achieve an ice-cream like consistency. You can play with your desired fruit to almond milk ratio depending on how thick you like it. Add sweetener to taste (we usually use super ripe bananas and find we don't need any). Top with hemp hearts, chia seeds, and unsweetened coconut flakes.

Enjoy!

Strawberry Banana Beet Ice Cream

Serves 1-2, as a dessert course

Ingredients:

- 1 frozen banana (freeze when very ripe)
- 1 cup frozen strawberries
- 1/2 of a beet
- Unsweetened almond milk, enough to blend
- Splash sweetener, if desired
- Hemp hearts
- Chia Seeds
- Cacao nibs
- Unsweetened coconut flakes

Directions:

1. Slice very ripe bananas and place in freezer along with the strawberries, preferably overnight.

2. Pour a generous splash of the almond milk into the blender (you will need to use more if you are not using a high speed blender). Throw in the frozen banana, frozen strawberries, and beet. Blend until you achieve an ice-cream like consistency. You can play with your desired fruit to almond milk ratio depending on how

thick you like it. Add sweetener to taste (we usually find that we don't need any). Top with hemp hearts, chia seeds, cacao nibs, and unsweetened coconut flakes.

Enjoy!

Moroccan Chickpea and Vegetable Tagine

Serves 3-4, as a main course

Ingredients:

- 2 tbsps coconut oil
- 1 onion
- 1 large clove of garlic
- 1 tbsp cumin
- 1 tbsp coriander
- 1/2 tbsp paprika
- 1 tbsp cinnamon
- 1/2 tsp sumac
- A pinch of fresh chilli
- 1 tbsp fresh ginger root
- 2 carrots, chopped into small rounds

- 1 sweet potato, skin on, chopped into medium sized cubes
- 1 large aubergine chopped into medium sized cubes
- 1 can/carton of drained and rinsed chickpeas
- 1 jar of tomato passata (680g) or two cans of chopped tomatoes
- 3 cups of water
- A handful of fresh dates, chopped roughly
- A handful each of fresh coriander and parsley

Directions:

1. Heat the coconut oil in a large pot, meanwhile chop the onion and garlic. Add the onion and garlic to the pot and cook on a medium heat with the lid on, so they can sweat and soften. After a few minutes, add the cumin, coriander, sumac, paprika, cinnamon, chilli and ginger and toast the spices for a few minutes to bring out the flavours until aromatic. Add around 1 1/2-2 cups of water, the passata and your chopped carrots and sweet potato and simmer for approximately 20 minutes, or until the vegetables are slightly soft when you stab them with a knife. Add the chopped aubergine and cook for a further 10 minutes, then add the

chickpeas, a handful of chopped fresh dates and a handful each of chopped fresh coriander and parsley. Mix well and allow it all to combine, adding the remaining water to thin it out a little. Serve topped with more fresh herbs and some rice or quinoa on the side, and keep the leftovers in the fridge for easy weeknight meals

Raw Vegan Pecan Pie

Serves 6-8, as a dessert course

Ingredients:

For the Base:

- 1 1/4 cup Oats (I use gluten free)
- 1/4 cup Water
- 3 fresh Dates
- 1 tsp Cinnamon

For the Caramel:

- 1 1/2 cups fresh dates
- 3 tbsps almond milk
- 2 tbsp Coconut oil

- 1/2 cup pecans to decorate

Directions:

1. For the base, simply combine all the ingredients in a food processor until it makes a moist but crumbly dough. Line a pie dish approximately 20cm in diameter with cling wrap and press the base mixture into it evenly. Place in the freezer to set, then get to work on the caramel. Clean the food processor bowl, then process the caramel ingredients until it makes a thick and gooey sauce. Spread it evenly over the frozen base, and press the pecans into it. Place it back into the freezer to set, then defrost slices whenever you want to eat it!

Quinoa Lentil Pumpkin Salad

Serves 4, as a main course

Ingredients:

- 150g quinoa (+350ml water)
- 100g red lentils (+250ml water)
- 2 large carrots
- ½ Hokkaido pumpkin
- 50g baby spinach
- olive oil for roasting
- handful of walnuts

Directions:

1. Cook quinoa and red lentils in two different sauce pans, adding more water if necessary. The lentils will need about 7-10 minutes, the quinoa approximately 15 minutes. Meanwhile cut the carrots and half of a Hokkaido pumpkin in smaller pieces and roast them in a pan and in olive oil at medium heat for 10 minutes. Wash the baby spinach and roughly shred it, using your hands. Mix all ingredients together in a big bowl and combine.

Farmer's Market Salad

Serves 2 to 4 , as a main course

Ingredients:

- 2 cups sliced zucchini and or summer squash
- 1 cup yellow wax beans, chopped in 2 inch pieces
- 1 cup sugar snap peas, trimmed
- 1 cup sliced radishes (¼ inch slices)
- ½ a kohlrabi, halved and sliced in ¼ inch slices
- 1 cup herb sprigs and leaves—flat leaf parsley, dill and basil
- 1 spring onion, thinly sliced
- Pinch chopped chives
- 2 tablespoons toasted sunflower seeds

Dressing

- 2 tablespoons flax oil
- 2 teaspoons apple cider vinegar
- 1 teaspoon tamari, plus more to taste
- Pinch flaky sea salt

Directions:

1. Seam vegetables in batches. Zucchini, wax beans, radishes and kohlrabi can be steamed for 2 minutes

each or until heated through, yet still crisp. Remove from steamer and spread out over a platter, wide bowl or a plate to cool. Steam sugar snap peas for one minute and add to vegetables. Set aside to cool completely before placing in a bowl and tossing with herbs, spring onions, chives and toasted sunflower seeds.

2. Stir the dressing ingredients together and drizzle over vegetables. Toss in any desired add ins and serve immediately.

Optional add ins;

- 1 cup cooked chickpeas or other beans
- Chopped avocado
- Thinly sliced kale
- Crumbled goat milk feta

Poached Halibut with Sweet Garlic, Parsley, and Lemon

Serves 2, as a main course

Ingredients:

- 4 cloves garlic, peeled and crushed
- 8 branches italian parsley
- 1 tsp salt
- Water
- 2 (~6-oz.) halibut fillets, skin removed, or another firm, white-fleshed fish such as cod, tilapia, or catfish
- Additional italian parsley branches, for garnish
- 2-4 juicy lemon wedges, for garnish
- Good-tasting extra-virgin olive oil, for serving
- Salt
- pepper

Directions:

1. Place the garlic, Italian parsley, and salt in a 12-inch skillet or sauté pan. Add water to a depth of about 2 inches. Bring to a simmer, cover, and let cook for 5 minutes. It should smell very fragrant.

2. Meanwhile, measure the thickness of the halibut fillets. They will cook for 8 to 10 minutes per inch of thickness.

3. When the poaching liquid is ready, slip the fillets gently into the pan. Cook for 8 to 10 minutes per inch, adjusting the heat so that the liquid just trembles: it should only bubble a little, and very gently. To test the fish for doneness, make a small slit with a paring knife in the thickest part of the fillet: all but the very center of each piece should be opaque.

4. When each fillet is ready, use a slotted spatula to transfer it to a serving plate. Garnish the plates with sprigs of Italian parsley and lemon wedges. Serve immediately, allowing each eater to season their fish at the table with olive oil, salt, pepper, and freshly squeezed lemon.

Raw Cauliflower Couscous with Kale and Cabbage

Serves 4, as a main course

Ingredients:

- ½ head cauliflower, grated (4 cups)
- 2 cups red cabbage, thinly sliced
- 2 cups tightly packed dino kale, thinly sliced*
- 5 stalks green onion, chopped (3/4 cup)
- 1 cup dried cranberries
- 1 cup raw walnuts, chopped
- 2 tablespoons olive oil
- ¼ cup fresh lemon juice
- 2 tablespoons stone ground mustard
- Salt and cracked pepper to taste

Directions:

1. Rinse all of the vegetables very well and pat dry.
2. Remove the stems on the cauliflower, chop the head in half, and grate one of the halves using a box grater (note: you can also pulse cauliflower florets in a food processor).

3. Add cauliflower couscous, cabbage, kale, green onion, dried cranberries, and walnuts to a large serving bowl.

4. Whisk together the olive oil, lemon juice, and stone ground mustard together in a small bowl. Pour it over the veggies and toss everything together well.

5. Serve alongside your favorite entree.

Mushroom with Lentils

Serves 2, as a main course

Ingredients:

- 3-4 tablespoons butter
- 4 large field or portabello mushrooms, sliced
- 250g (9oz) cooked lentils
- 1-2 tablespoons tomato paste
- 1 bunch flat leaf parsley, leaves picked

Directions:

1. Heat butter over a medium heat in a large frying pan. Add mushrooms and cook, stirring every few minutes or until mushrooms are browned and tender. About 10 minutes.

2. Add lentils and tomato paste and cook until warm.

3. Taste. Season and serve with parsley on top.

VARIATIONS

short on time? – use a drained can of lentils instead of cooking your own.

vegan / dairy-free – replace butter with coconut oil or olive oil.

need help cooking your lentils? – just simmer like pasta until tender. Depending on the type of lentil it will take from 15-30 minutes.

paleo / lentil-free – replace lentils with minced (ground) beef – make sure it's well browned and cooked through before serving.

different veg / mushroom-free – replace mushies with eggplant (aubergine), kale, broccoli brussels sprouts – whatever you feel like really.

Avocado Tofu Salad with Ponzu Recipe

Serves 4, as a main course

Ingredients:

- 1 large avocado, firm, not too soft
- 7 ounces of extra firm tofu (1/2 of a standard package)
- 1 small Persian cucumber
- 3 Tablespoons ponzu sauce (Kikkoman's is fine or make your own)
- Salad greens, preferably baby lettuce
- 1 green onion, minced
- Toasted sesame seeds

Directions:

1. Slice the avocado in half, remove the pit, cut into medium size chunks and place in a mixing bowl. Drain the tofu and cut into chunks, roughly the same size as the avocado. Add to the mixing bowl along with the ponzu sauce and toss, gently. Allow to marinate for at least 4 hours, preferably overnight. Use a mandolin to slice the cucumber into thin slices, or cut with a knife. Line each plate or bowl with salad greens, top them with cucumber slices. Place the avocado mixture on top

of the salad greens and top each serving with green onion and sesame seeds. Drizzle each serving with a bit of the ponzu sauce.

Pesto with Walnuts

Serves 4, as a other course

Ingredients:

- two handfulls fresh basil
- 6 garlic cloves
- 1/2 cup walnuts
- 1 tsp salt
- 1/2 tsp black pepper
- olive oil
- 1/2 cup grated parmesan cheese (optional)

Directions:

1. Grab your handy food processor and toss in the 6 peeled garlic cloves.
2. Blend until small pieces are sticking to the sides of the container.
3. Add washed basil leaves picked from the stems, walnuts, salt, pepper, and olive oil.

4. Blend and add olive oil if needed until mixture becomes a paste.

5. Scoop out the mixture into a bowl and stir in the grated parmesan (optional).

6. Serve mixed in with cooked pasta, smeared over pan-seared fish or shrimp, or spread inside a veggie pita.

Black Risotto

Serves 2-4, as a main course

Ingredients:

- 3 medium-sized fresh cuttlefish
- 3 medium-sized fresh squid
- 1/3 cup olive oil
- 1 large onion, finely chopped
- 4 cloves garlic, finely grated
- 3-4 tbsp chopped flat leaf parsley
- Salt & fresh cracked pepper, to taste
- ¼ cup red wine
- ¼ cup red wine vinegar
- 1 cup arborio rice

- 1 clove garlic, grated, plus ½ small onion finely chopped, plus 1 tbsp olive oil, extra
- Lemon slices and chopped parsley, to garnish

Directions:

1. To clean the cuttlefish: wash it well under running water. Tear through the back and discard the backbone and insides, carefully separating the small silvery ink sack and setting it aside. Peel the skin from the flesh and discard. Cut the tentacles just below the eyes, squeeze the beak out from the centre of the tentacles and discard. Set the tentacles to one side.

2. To clean the squid: basically follow the same method as the cuttlefish but tear off the two "wings" near the point. These can be eaten as well and all you need to do is peel the skin off them. Remember to set the tentacles aside with the ones from the cuttlefish. Keep all the ink sacks in a little dish on the side.

3. Slice the cuttlefish and squid into approximate 2cm x 4cm strips. To extract the ink, break the sacks and squeeze out the paste. Add a few drops of water to make it a smooth consistency.

4. Heat a large saucepan with the 1/3 cup olive oil over medium heat. Sauté the large chopped onion and when soft, add the sliced cuttlefish and squid, not the tentacles, and cook until lightly golden. Add the 4 cloves garlic and chopped parsley, stirring to combine. Pour in the wine, vinegar and then stir in the ink paste. Cook for a further 5 minutes. Season with salt and pepper, to taste.

5. Add the rice to the saucepan along with an extra tablespoon of oil. Stir the rice into the seafood and sauté for 1-2 minutes. Add enough hot water to cover the rice completely, reduce heat to low and cook, uncovered, until rice is al dente. Stir occasionally. If the rice dries out before it is cooked just add small amounts of hot water each time, stirring, until cooked. Do not let it stick!

6. In a separate small frying pan heat the extra tablespoon of oil and sauté the chopped ½ onion over medium heat until soft. Add the reserved tentacles and garlic and sauté for 1-2 minutes. Throw in a little chopped parsley and salt.

7. To serve, dish up the risotto in individual bowls, top with the sautéed tentacles, more parsley and a cheek

of fresh lemon. A side salad of fresh leaves, glass of vino and crusty bread wouldn't go astray, either.

Quinoa Carrot Cakes

Serves 10, as a dessert course

Ingredients:

- 1/2 cup apple juice
- 4 tbsp brown rice syrup or honey
- 3 tbsp milled flaxseed
- 2 tbsp extra virgin olive oil
- 1 cup grated carrots
- pinch of sea salt
- 1/2 cup quinoa flour
- 3/4 cup brown rice flour (plain gluten-free flour will work)
- 2 tsp baking powder
- 2 tsp cinnamon
- 1 tbsp rapadura or coconut sugar (optional topping)
- 1/4 tsp cinnamon (topping)

Directions:

1. Preheat the oven to 180°Celsius, 160°C fan assisted or 350°Fahrenheit. Line a generous muffin tray with 10 paper cases.

2. In a large bowl, mix the apricots, banana, walnuts, apple juice, honey, flaxseed and oil. Stir through the grated carrots and salt. Set aside.

3. In a separate bowl, sieve the flour with the baking powder and cinnamon. Make sure the baking powder doesn't stick in one place. Make a well in the centre of the flour and scoop the wet mixture into it. Spoon the dough into your cupcake liners. You're aiming for exactly 10 cupcakes.

4. Bake for 40 minutes. Remove from the oven and let your nostrils dance. Now stir the coconut sugar and cinnamon together, sprinkling over each cupcake.

Arugula and Lentil Salad with Strawberry-Balsamic Dressing

Serves 6, as a salad course

Ingredients:

For the salad:

- 6-8 cups fresh arugula
    - 1.5 cups cooked lentils (~3/4 cup dry)
- 1 cup fresh strawberries, sliced
- 3 garlic scapes, finely minced (or green onions / scallions)
- 1 cup fromage frais (or cottage cheese or ricotta) - optional, omit for a vegan salad
- 1/2 cup sliced almonds, toasted
- 2 tbsp fresh basil leaves, chiffonade

strawberry-Balsamic Dressing (yields ~1.5 cups):

- 1.5 cups fresh strawberries
- 2 tbsp balsamic vinegar
- 1/4 cup water
- 1/4 cup flaxseed oil
- 1 tbsp fresh basil
- Pinch of salt

Directions:

1. If not already done, first cook the lentils. In a medium pot, bring 2 cups of water, a pinch of salt and the lentils to a boil. Reduce heat and simmer for 25 minutes. Drain any excess water and set aside.

2. Dry toast the almonds over medium heat for a few minutes until golden. Set aside.

3. For the dressing: In the measuring beaker that came with your hand blender (or in a mason jar), add the strawberries, balsamic vinegar, water, flaxseed oil, basil leaves and a pinch of salt.

4. Process the dressing until nice and smooth. Refrigerate until ready to serve. This can be done a few hours (up to one day) ahead of time.

5. To assemble the salad: Place a large handful of arugula on each plate. Sprinkle ~1/4 cup cooked lentils, a generous pinch of minced garlic scapes and decorate with fresh strawberry pieces.

6. Top with fromage frais if using, and sprinkle the toasted almonds and basil chiffonade over each plate.

7. Pour the strawberry-balsamic dressing over the salad and savour at once.

Creamy Mango and Rhubarb Smoothie

Serves 1-2, as a beverage course

Ingredients:

- 1 ripe mango, peeled, pitted and diced
- 1 and 1/2 cup diced rhubarb (~ 3 thin stalks)
- 1/2 cup cashews, soaked in water overnight and drained (prior soaking is optional)
- 1 cup soy milk
- 1/2 cup water
- A squeeze of lime juice
- A drop of pure vanilla extract

Directions:

1. In a blender or a 1-quart mason jar (if using an immersion blender), add the mango, rhubarb, drained cashews, soy milk, water, a squeeze of lime juice and a drop of vanilla extract.
2. Process until very smooth. If you prefer a thinner smoothie, add more soy milk or water. Serve topped with thin slices of raw rhubarb and a sprig of fresh mint.

3. Note: You could, of course, freeze the diced mango and rhubarb for a couple of hours prior to blending.

Zesty Orange and Carrot Smoothie

Serves 1-2, as a beverage course

Ingredients:

- 2 small oranges, peeled and sliced or segmented
- 2 small carrots, sliced
- 1-inch piece of fresh ginger, roughly chopped
- 2 cups water
- 1 tsp maple syrup (optional)
- 1 tsp maca powder (optional)
- 1/2 tsp turmeric powder (optional)

Directions:

1. Combine all ingredients into a blender.
2. Process until smooth.
3. Yields one large or two small servings.

Roasted baby cauliflower, fried coriander chickpeas, caper dressing, crushed pistachio and greek yogurt

Serves 1-3, as a main course

Ingredients:

- 5 tablespoons olive oil, divided
- 1lb. purple baby cauliflower, de-stemmed
- 1 (14oz.) can of chickpeas, drained
- 1 teaspoon coriander
- 1/4 cup greek yogurt
- 1 lemon, juice + zest
- 1/4 cup crushed pistachios
- Sea salt to taste
- Freshly ground pepper

caper Dressing:

- 2 tbsp capers, drained
- 1 garlic clove, minced
- 1 lemon, juice
- 3-4 fresh mint leaves
- Sea salt to taste
- Freshly ground pepper

Directions:

1. Preheat oven to 400 degrees. Drizzle about 2 tablespoons of olive oil on a large baking sheet. Add cauliflower to the pan, flipping to make sure they are coated on both sides. Squeeze the juice of one lemon over the baby cauliflower. Season with sea salt and roast for 30-35 minutes or until browned and tender.

2. In a small mason jar, muddle capers garlic and mint leaves together. Squeeze in lemon juice and season to taste with sea salt and pepper. Drizzle in a few tablespoons of olive oil until your desired consistency. Screw on mason jar lid and shake until well combined.

3. In a small mixing bowl, whisk together coriander with sea salt and freshly ground pepper to taste. Set aside

4. In a skillet, coat pan with 2-3 tablespoons of olive oil. Over medium-high heat, drop in chickpeas in batches, frying until golden and charred. While chickpeas are hot, sprinkle a generous amount of coriander seasoning. Place chickpeas on a paper towel-lined plate to soak up excess oil. Continue frying in batches until all chickpeas are fried and seasoned.

5. To plate, smear a few tablespoons of greek yogurt before topping with whole cauliflower and fried

chickpeas. Drizzle caper dressing generously over top. Garnish with crushed pistachios, sea salt, freshly ground pepper and fresh mint leaves.

Eat to Beat Brownies

Serves 1-10, as a dessert course

Ingredients:

- ¾ cup gluten free oats (you can put in a food processor- however, I like mine chewy so I keep them whole)
- ½ cup Justin's Vanilla almond Butter (personal favorite)
- ½ cup dark chocolate chips (I use Lily's dark chocolate baking chips which are vegan, fair-trade, organic and have no sugar added)
- ½ cup unsweetened cocoa powder (non-alkalized)
- ½ cup unsweetened apple cinnamon applesauce
- ¼ cup honey
- 1 ½ cup shredded zucchini (needs to be patted very dry or your brownies will have too much liquid)

- ¼ cup shredded carrot (needs to be patted very dry as well)
- 1 tsp vanilla
- 2 tsp cinnamon
- 1 tsp baking soda
- Your choice of: chopped nuts (i.e. walnuts), chopped dried fruit (i.e. dried cherries), flax seed, or all of the above (my preference).

Directions:

1. Preheat oven to 350 degrees F.
2. Blend oats in food processor, if desired. (Not necessary, I use them whole).
3. Combine all ingredients into a mixing bowl, saving the chocolate chips for last. (Use additional chocolate chips to sprinkle on top, if desired). Fold in the grated carrot and zucchini after patting completely dry on paper towels.
4. Pour batter into an 8x11 pan and bake for 25-30 minutes. Enjoy!

Indian Spiced Tomato Soup

8, as a soup course

Ingredients:

- 1 c. short grain brown rice
- 2 T. butter or olive oil
- 1 large yellow onion, diced
- 1 tsp. sea salt
- 3 tsp. curry powder
- 1 tsp. coriander seeds
- 1 tsp. cumin seeds
- 1/2 tsp. red pepper flakes
- 2 28 oz. cans of crushed tomatoes
- 1 14 oz. can of coconut milk
- 1/2 c. sliced almonds
- 1/2 c. tightly packed cilantro leaves, chopped

Directions:

1. Place the rice in a medium sized heavy bottomed pot (set aside your biggest pot for the soup). Pour in 2 cups of water, cover and bring to a boil. Turn down the heat as low as it will go and simmer, covered for 45 minutes, or until all the liquid has evaporated.

2. Meanwhile, melt the butter in the big pot over medium heat. Add the onions and cool until translucent, 8-10 minutes. Add the spices, stir to coat the onions, and cook for 1 minute. Add the tomatoes and 6 cups of water, cover, and bring to a boil. Turn to medium low and simmer, covered, until everything is cooked down. I just cooked it until the rice was almost done. Puree with a hand blender, then stir in the coconut milk.
3. While the rice is cooking, place the almonds in a dry skillet and heat on medium until browned and fragrant, stirring occasionally.
4. Serve soup with a scoop of rice, some toasted almonds and a sprinkling of cilantro.

Spiced Chocolate Mousse

Serves 1-4, as a dessert course

Ingredients:

- 3-4 Tablespoons maple syrup
- 2 Ripe Avocados
- 2 Teaspoons Of Tamari (A Wheat-Free Soya Sauce)
- 6 Tablespoons Cocoa or Cacao Powder
- 2 Tablespoons Cashew, Hazelnut or Macadamia Butter
- ½ Teaspoon Cinnamon
- ¼ Teaspoon Cayenne Pepper (for heat, not sting)
- 1 Teaspoon Ginger Juice (or ¼ Teaspoon dried Ginger)
- Seeds From 1/4 Pomegranate
- Coconut Yoghurt

Directions:

1. Pulse all ingredients with a handheld blender, divide into small glass tumblers, and refigerate for 30 minutes. Top with coconut milk yogurt and pomegranate seeds.

Baked Tarragon Oil & Lemon Fish with Kale Pesto Quinoa

Serves 4, as a main course

Ingredients:

Kale Pesto:

- 1/2 cup almonds
- 2 tablespoons walnut oil
- 2 garlic cloves, roughly chopped
- 1/3 cup parmesan
- 4-5 kale leaves, de-stemmed and roughly chopped
- Extra Virgin Olive Oil

Tarragon Oil:

- 1/2 cup + 3 tablespoons olive oil
- 1 oz. fresh tarragon
- 1lb. whitefish, (we used Pollock)
- 2 meyer lemons, sliced in rounds
- Sea salt to taste
- Freshly ground pepper
- 1 cup quinoa

Directions:

1. Serve this meal warm with a lemon wedge and season with sea salt and freshly ground pepper. For detailed directions on how to make this recipe, please visit the site of our generous contributor sassy-kitchen.

Roasted Spiced Chickpeas Over Kale Caesar Salad

Serves 1-4, as a salad course

Ingredients:

chickpeas:

- 1 can chickpeas, drained
- 1/4 cup sesame seeds
- 3 tablespoons olive oil
- 1 teaspoon cumin
- 1 teaspon garlic powder
- 1 teaspoon sea salt
- 1/2 teaspoon coriander
- 1/2 teaspoon cayenne
- 1/2 teaspoon paprika

- 1/2 teaspoon fresh ground pepper
- 1/4 teaspoon turmeric

Salad:

- 3/4 cup cashews, raw
- 1 teaspoon yellow miso
- 1/2 teaspoon apple cider vinegar
- 2 garlic cloves, whole
- 2 teaspoons lemon juice
- 1 teaspoon nori, chopped
- 1 teaspoon nutritional yeast
- 2 tablespoons coconut cream
- 1/2 cup water
- 1 teaspoon tamari, gluten-free
- 1/2 teaspoon black pepper
- 1 teaspoon sea salt
- 1 head of kale, de-stremmed and chopped
- 1/2 avocado, diced

Directions:

For the chickpeas:

1. Preheat oven to 400 degrees. Add drained chickpeas to a large mixing bowl. Mix in all spices, sesame seeds

and olive oil with sea salt and pepper. Use your hands to make sure chickpeas are evenly coated with mixture. Roast for 40-45 minutes or until crisp and browned. Set aside to cool.

For the salad:

1. Add the first twelve ingredients to a blender or food processor and blend until smooth. In a large bowl, add kale, avocado and dresssing. Mix together with your hands until well combine. Top with roasted chickpeas and enjoy!

Roasted Beet Pesto

Serves variant, as a spread course

Ingredients:

- 1 cup red beets, chopped and roasted (about 1 medium beet)
- 3 cloves garlic, roughly chopped
- ½ cup walnuts, roasted
- ½ cup parmesan cheese, grated
- ½ cup olive oil
- 2 tablespoons lemon juice
- Salt to taste

Directions:

1. Preheat the oven to 375 degrees F.
2. Wash and scrub the beet and pat it dry. Chop it into ½" cubes and place it on a sheet of foil. Wrap the chopped beet in foil, making a foil packet.
3. Place the packet on a baking sheet.
4. Roast in the oven for 50 minutes, or until beets are soft and juices are seeping out.
5. Allow beets to cool completely.

6. Add all ingredients except for the oil to a food processor or blender and pulse several times.

7. Leaving the food processor (or blender) running, slowly add the olive oil until all ingredients are well combined. If the pesto is too thick for your blender to process, add a small amount of water until desired consistency is reached.

Sweet Potato Apple Soup

Serves 6-8, as a soup course

Ingredients:

- 2 tablespoons olive oil
- 2 large sweet potatos peeled and chopped
- 2-3 carrots peeled and chopped
- 1 apple cored and chopped
- 1 onion chopped
- 1 garlic crushed
- 1/2 cup red lentils
- 1/4 tsp ginger to taste) fresh or dried
- 1/2 tsp cumin
- 1/2 tsp chili powder

- 1/2 tsp paprika
- salt to taste
- 4 cups vegetable broth
- sprigs of thyme and plain yogurt for garnish

Directions:

1. Melt margarine over medium-high heat. Place the chopped potatoes, carrots, apple, garlic and onion. Cook until onion translucent.
2. Stir in lentils, and seasoning and add broth. Bring the soup to boil over high heat and then reduce and simmer until lentil and vegetable are soft. (30 minutes)
3. Pour the soup in a blender in batches and puree. Be careful not to over blend. Return to pan to maintain temperature. If desired serve with a dab or yogurt and ginger, garnish with thyme.

Pecan, Granny Smith & Kale salad

Serves Serves 2, as a side course

Ingredients:

- 2 cups finely chopped kale
- 1/8 cup chopped pecans
- 1/8 cup chopped celery
- 1 chopped granny smith apple
- 1/2 cup shredded red cabbage
- 2 tablespoons orange juice
- 2 tablespoons lemon juice
- 1/2 tsp. chopped chives or 1/4 tsp. onion powder
- 1/2 tsp. garlic powder or 1 small garlic clove chopped
- 1/4 teaspoon dried parsley
- 1/4 tsp. ground flaxseed

...Pairs well with grilled salmon!

Directions:

1. Chop kale, pecans, celery, apple. chives and garlic (unless using powdered herbs)
2. Squeeze orange and lemon juice.
3. Place apples in bowl first and blend with juice.
4. Mix in all remaining ingredients, including herbs.

5. Serve

Has a nice tartness and crunch that pairs nicely with grilled salmon or a creamy pumpkin or butternut squash soup.

100% of ingredients have anti-angiogenic properties and can be served in a matter of minutes.

Give each family member 1-2 things to squeeze or chop and voila in mere minutes a delicious, anti-angiogenesis meal appears.

Sweet Potato and Turnip Mash with Fresh Sage

Serves 6, as a side course

Ingredients:

- 1 pound sweet potatoes, peeled and diced
- 8 ounces turnips (about 2 medium), peeled and diced
- 3 large cloves garlic
- 20 fresh sage leaves, divided (8 left whole, the rest cut into strips)
- 2 tablespoons olive oil
- 1 teaspoon kosher or sea salt

- ½ teaspoon coarsely cracked pepper

Directions:

1. Place potatoes, turnips, garlic and 8 sage leaves in a medium saucepan and cover with water. Bring to a boil. Reduce the heat to medium-low, cover, and simmer until the vegetables are fork-tender, 12 to 15 minutes. Drain. Return the vegetables to the pan and keep covered.
2. Heat butter in a small skillet over medium-high heat. As it melts and turns lightly brown, add the olive oil and strips of sage and allow them to crackle and flavor the butter, about 1 minute.
3. Pour the sage and olive oil over the vegetables and smash with a potato masher. Stir in salt and pepper and serve.

Sauteed Chicken Breast with Kale and Wild Mushrooms

Serves 4-6, as a main course

Ingredients:

- 1 pound kale, tough stems discarded, leaves cut into 2-inch pieces
- 1 tablespoon all-purpose flour
- 2 teaspoons unsalted butter, softened
- 1 tablespoon plus 2 teaspoons extra-virgin olive oil
- Four 6-ounce skinless, boneless chicken breast halves, lightly pounded
- Salt and freshly ground black pepper
- ½ pound wild mushrooms, such as oyster mushrooms or chanterelle, sliced ⅓-inch thick
- 3 medium shallots, minced
- ⅓ cup dry white wine
- ⅔ cup chicken stock or canned low-sodium broth
- 2 teaspoons fresh lemon juice

Directions:

1. Blanch the kale in a large pot of salted water until limp, about 2 minutes. Drain well, pressing to extract excess

water. In a small bowl, blend the flour and butter until smooth.

2. Heat 1 teaspoon of the oil in the skillet. Season the chicken with salt and pepper. Add the breasts to the skillet and cook over moderately high heat until brown and crusty on the bottom, about 4 minutes. Turn and cook the other side until lightly browned, about 3 minutes. Transfer the chicken to a platter and cover loosely with foil.

3. Heat 1 teaspoon of the oil in the skillet. Add the mushrooms, shallots and 2 tablespoons of water, season with salt and pepper and cook over moderate heat, stirring occasionally, until the vegetables are softened and browned, about 6 minutes. Transfer to a bowl and keep warm.

4. Pour the wine into the skillet and cook over high heat, scraping the bottom of the pan to loosen any browned bits, until reduced to a few tablespoons. Add the chicken stock and cook until reduced to 1/2 cup, about 3 minutes. Whisk in the flour paste and cook until the sauce thickens. Add the mushrooms and cook until warmed through. Transfer to a small bowl and stir in any accumulated juices from the chicken.

5. Wipe out the skillet and return it to high heat. Add the remaining 1 teaspoon oil . Add the kale, season with salt and pepper and sauté until just beginning to brown, about 3 minutes. Stir in the lemon juice. Arrange the kale on 4 dinner plates. Top with the chicken breasts and mushroom sauce and serve.

Serve With Gluten Free Quinoa

Made in the USA
Monee, IL
21 June 2021

71910760R00046